VETERINARY
CONTROLLED SUBSTANCE
LOG BOOK

NAME _____

_____

ADDRESS _____

_____

EMAIL _____

PHONE NUMBER _____

LOG BOOK DETAILS

LOG START DATE _____

LOG END DATE _____

LOG BOOK NUMBER _____

NOTES: ....

....

....

....

....

CONTROLLED SUBSTANCE: .... STRENGTH: .... FROM: ....

DATE	CLIENT, PATIENT	ADDRESS/ID/SERIAL #	UNIQUE BOTTE #	REASON NOTES	ADMIN/ DISPENSED BY:	AMOUNT OF/ WASTE/ HUB LOSS	AMOUNT ADDED	AMOUNT USED	ENDING BALANCE
				☐ BEGINNING BALANCE OR	☐ BALANCE FROM PREVIOUS PAGE	⇧			

DATE	CLIENT, PATIENT	ADDRESS/ID/SERIAL #	UNIQUE BOTTLE #	REASON NOTES	ADMIN/ DISPENSED BY:	AMOUNT OF/ WASTE/ HUB LOSS	AMOUNT ADDED	AMOUNT USED	ENDING BALANCE
				☐ BEGINNING BALANCE OR		☐ BALANCE FROM PREVIOUS PAGE		⇧	

CONTROLLED SUBSTANCE: .... STRENGTH: .... FROM: ....

DATE	CLIENT, PATIENT	ADDRESS/ID/SERIAL #	UNIQUE BOTTLE #	REASON NOTES	ADMIN/ DISPENSED BY:	AMOUNT OF/ WASTE/ HUB LOSS	AMOUNT ADDED	AMOUNT USED	ENDING BALANCE
				☐ BEGINNING BALANCE OR		☐ BALANCE FROM PREVIOUS PAGE		⇧	

DATE	CLIENT, PATIENT	ADDRESS/ID/SERIAL #	UNIQUE BOTTLE #	REASON NOTES	ADMIN/ DISPENSED BY:	AMOUNT OF/ WASTE/ HUB LOSS	AMOUNT ADDED	AMOUNT USED	ENDING BALANCE
						☐ BALANCE FROM PREVIOUS PAGE ⇧			
					☐ BEGINNING BALANCE OR				

CONTROLLED SUBSTANCE: .... STRENGTH: .... FROM: ....

DATE	CLIENT, PATIENT	ADDRESS/ID/SERIAL #	UNIQUE BOTTLE #	REASON NOTES	ADMIN/ DISPENSED BY:	AMOUNT OF/ WASTE/ HUB LOSS	AMOUNT ADDED	AMOUNT USED	ENDING BALANCE
				☐ BEGINNING BALANCE OR		☐ BALANCE FROM PREVIOUS PAGE		⇧	

CONTROLLED SUBSTANCE:

STRENGTH:

FORM:

DATE	CLIENT, PATIENT	ADDRESS/ID/SERIAL #	UNIQUE BOTTE #	REASON NOTES	ADMIN/ DISPENSED BY:	AMOUNT OF/ WASTE/ HUB LOSS	AMOUNT ADDED	AMOUNT USED	ENDING BALANCE
				☐ BEGINNING BALANCE OR		☐ BALANCE FROM PREVIOUS PAGE ⇧			

CONTROLLED SUBSTANCE: .... STRENGTH: .... FROM: ....

DATE	CLIENT, PATIENT	ADDRESS/ID/SERIAL #	UNIQUE BOTTLE #	REASON NOTES	ADMIN/ DISPENSED BY:	AMOUNT OF/ WASTE/ HUB LOSS	AMOUNT ADDED	AMOUNT USED	ENDING BALANCE
				☐ BEGINNING BALANCE OR		☐ BALANCE FROM PREVIOUS PAGE		⇧	

DATE	CLIENT, PATIENT	ADDRESS/ID/SERIAL #	UNIQUE BOTTE #	REASON NOTES	ADMIN/ DISPENSED BY:	AMOUNT OF/ WASTE/ HUB LOSS	AMOUNT ADDED	AMOUNT USED	ENDING BALANCE
				☐ BEGINNING BALANCE OR		☐ BALANCE FROM PREVIOUS PAGE		⇧	

CONTROLLED SUBSTANCE: .... STRENGTH: .... FROM: ....

DATE	CLIENT, PATIENT	ADDRESS/ID/SERIAL #	UNIQUE BOTTLE #	REASON NOTES	ADMIN/ DISPENSED BY:	AMOUNT OF/ WASTE/ HUB LOSS	AMOUNT ADDED	AMOUNT USED	ENDING BALANCE
				☐ BEGINNING BALANCE OR		☐ BALANCE FROM PREVIOUS PAGE ⇦			

CONTROLLED SUBSTANCE: _____ STRENGTH: _____ FROM: _____

DATE	CLIENT, PATIENT	ADDRESS/ID/SERIAL #	UNIQUE BOTTLE #	REASON NOTES	ADMIN/ DISPENSED BY:	AMOUNT OF/ WASTE/ HUB LOSS	AMOUNT ADDED	AMOUNT USED	ENDING BALANCE
				☐ BEGINNING BALANCE OR		☐ BALANCE FROM PREVIOUS PAGE		⇧	

CONTROLLED SUBSTANCE: ....

STRENGTH: ....

FROM: ....

DATE	CLIENT, PATIENT	ADDRESS/ID/SERIAL #	UNIQUE BOTTE #	REASON NOTES	ADMIN/ DISPENSED BY:	AMOUNT OF/ WASTE/ HUB LOSS	AMOUNT ADDED	AMOUNT USED	ENDING BALANCE
				☐ BEGINNING BALANCE OR		☐ BALANCE FROM PREVIOUS PAGE		⇧	

DATE	CLIENT, PATIENT	ADDRESS/ID/SERIAL #	UNIQUE BOTTLE #	REASON NOTES	ADMIN/ DISPENSED BY:	AMOUNT OF/ WASTE/ HUB LOSS	AMOUNT ADDED	AMOUNT USED	ENDING BALANCE
				□ BEGINNING BALANCE OR		□ BALANCE FROM PREVIOUS PAGE		⇦	

CONTROLLED SUBSTANCE: ....

STRENGTH: ....

FROM: ....

DATE	CLIENT, PATIENT	ADDRESS/ID/SERIAL #	UNIQUE BOTTLE #	REASON NOTES	ADMIN/ DISPENSED BY:	AMOUNT OF/ WASTE/ HUB LOSS	AMOUNT ADDED	AMOUNT USED	ENDING BALANCE
				☐ BEGINNING BALANCE OR	☐ BALANCE FROM PREVIOUS PAGE ⇧				

CONTROLLED SUBSTANCE: _____ STRENGTH: _____ FROM: _____

DATE	CLIENT. PATIENT	ADDRESS/ID/SERIAL #	UNIQUE BOTTE #	REASON NOTES	ADMIN/ DISPENSED BY:	AMOUNT OF/ WASTE/ HUB LOSS	AMOUNT ADDED	AMOUNT USED	ENDING BALANCE
				☐ BEGINNING BALANCE OR		☐ BALANCE FROM PREVIOUS PAGE		⇧	

CONTROLLED SUBSTANCE: ....   STRENGTH: ....   FROM: ....

DATE	CLIENT, PATIENT	ADDRESS/ID/SERIAL #	UNIQUE BOTTLE #	REASON NOTES	ADMIN/ DISPENSED BY:	AMOUNT OF/ WASTE/ HUB LOSS	AMOUNT ADDED	AMOUNT USED	ENDING BALANCE
				☐ BEGINNING BALANCE OR		☐ BALANCE FROM PREVIOUS PAGE		⬆	

DATE	CLIENT, PATIENT	ADDRESS/ID/SERIAL #	UNIQUE BOTTE #	REASON NOTES	ADMIN/ DISPENSED BY:	AMOUNT OF/ WASTE/ HUB LOSS	AMOUNT ADDED	AMOUNT USED	ENDING BALANCE
				☐ BEGINNING BALANCE OR	☐ BALANCE FROM PREVIOUS PAGE ⇧				

CONTROLLED SUBSTANCE: .... STRENGTH: .... FROM: ....

DATE	CLIENT, PATIENT	ADDRESS/ID/SERIAL #	UNIQUE BOTTE #	REASON NOTES	ADMIN/ DISPENSED BY:	AMOUNT OF/ WASTE/ HUB LOSS	AMOUNT ADDED	AMOUNT USED	ENDING BALANCE
				☐ BEGINNING BALANCE OR		☐ BALANCE FROM PREVIOUS PAGE ⇧			

CONTROLLED SUBSTANCE: _____ STRENGTH: _____ FROM: _____

DATE	CLIENT. PATIENT	ADDRESS/ID/SERIAL #	UNIQUE BOTTLE #	REASON NOTES	ADMIN/ DISPENSED BY:	AMOUNT OF/ WASTE/ HUB LOSS	AMOUNT ADDED	AMOUNT USED	ENDING BALANCE
				☐ BEGINNING BALANCE OR ☐ BALANCE FROM PREVIOUS PAGE				⇧	

CONTROLLED SUBSTANCE: .... STRENGTH: .... FROM: ....

DATE	CLIENT, PATIENT	ADDRESS/ID/SERIAL #	UNIQUE BOTTE #	REASON NOTES	ADMIN/ DISPENSED BY:	AMOUNT OF/ WASTE/ HUB LOSS	AMOUNT ADDED	AMOUNT USED	ENDING BALANCE
				☐ BEGINNING BALANCE OR		☐ BALANCE FROM PREVIOUS PAGE	⇧	⇧	

DATE	CLIENT, PATIENT	ADDRESS/ID/SERIAL #	UNIQUE BOTTE #	REASON NOTES	ADMIN/ DISPENSED BY:	AMOUNT OF/ WASTE/ HUB LOSS	AMOUNT ADDED	AMOUNT USED	ENDING BALANCE
				☐ BEGINNING BALANCE OR		☐ BALANCE FROM PREVIOUS PAGE ⇧			

CONTROLLED SUBSTANCE: ---------- STRENGTH: ---------- FROM: ----------

DATE	CLIENT, PATIENT	ADDRESS/ID/SERIAL #	UNIQUE BOTTE #	REASON NOTES	ADMIN/ DISPENSED BY:	AMOUNT OF/ WASTE/ HUB LOSS	AMOUNT ADDED	AMOUNT USED	ENDING BALANCE
				☐ BEGINNING BALANCE OR		☐ BALANCE FROM PREVIOUS PAGE		⇧	

DATE	CLIENT, PATIENT	ADDRESS/ID/SERIAL #	UNIQUE BOTTLE #	REASON NOTES	ADMIN/ DISPENSED BY:	AMOUNT OF/ WASTE/ HUB LOSS	AMOUNT ADDED	AMOUNT USED	ENDING BALANCE
					☐ BEGINNING BALANCE OR	☐ BALANCE FROM PREVIOUS PAGE		⇧	

CONTROLLED SUBSTANCE: .... STRENGTH: .... FROM: ....

DATE	CLIENT, PATIENT	ADDRESS/ID/SERIAL #	UNIQUE BOTTE #	REASON NOTES	ADMIN/ DISPENSED BY:	AMOUNT OF/ WASTE/ HUB LOSS	AMOUNT ADDED	AMOUNT USED	ENDING BALANCE
				☐ BEGINNING BALANCE OR		☐ BALANCE FROM PREVIOUS PAGE		⇧	

DATE	CLIENT, PATIENT	ADDRESS/ID/SERIAL #	UNIQUE BOTTE #	REASON NOTES	ADMIN/ DISPENSED BY:	AMOUNT OF/ WASTE/ HUB LOSS	AMOUNT ADDED	AMOUNT USED	ENDING BALANCE
				☐ BEGINNING BALANCE OR	☐ BALANCE FROM PREVIOUS PAGE			⇧	

CONTROLLED SUBSTANCE: .... STRENGTH: .... FROM: ....

DATE	CLIENT, PATIENT	ADDRESS/ID/SERIAL #	UNIQUE BOTTLE #	REASON NOTES	ADMIN/ DISPENSED BY:	AMOUNT OF/ WASTE/ HUB LOSS	AMOUNT ADDED	AMOUNT USED	ENDING BALANCE
				☐ BEGINNING BALANCE OR	☐ BALANCE FROM PREVIOUS PAGE			⇧	

CONTROLLED SUBSTANCE ....

STRENGTH ...... FROM ..

DATE	CLIENT, PATIENT	ADDRESS/ID/SERIAL #	UNIQUE BOTTE #	REASON NOTES	ADMIN/ DISPENSED BY:	AMOUNT OF/ WASTE/ HUB LOSS	AMOUNT ADDED	AMOUNT USED	ENDING BALANCE
				☐ BEGINNING BALANCE OR	☐ BALANCE FROM PREVIOUS PAGE	⇧			

CONTROLLED SUBSTANCE: .... STRENGTH: .... FROM: ....

DATE	CLIENT, PATIENT	ADDRESS/ID/SERIAL #	UNIQUE BOTTLE #	REASON NOTES	ADMIN/ DISPENSED BY:	AMOUNT OF/ WASTE/ HUB LOSS	AMOUNT ADDED	AMOUNT USED	ENDING BALANCE
				☐ BEGINNING BALANCE OR		☐ BALANCE FROM PREVIOUS PAGE		⇧	

DATE	CLIENT, PATIENT	ADDRESS/ID/SERIAL #	UNIQUE BOTTE #	REASON NOTES	ADMIN/ DISPENSED BY:	AMOUNT OF/ WASTE/ HUB LOSS	AMOUNT ADDED	AMOUNT USED	ENDING BALANCE
						☐ BEGINNING BALANCE OR ☐ BALANCE FROM PREVIOUS PAGE ⇧			

CONTROLLED SUBSTANCE: ....

STRENGTH: ....   FROM: ....

DATE	CLIENT, PATIENT	ADDRESS/ID/SERIAL #	UNIQUE BOTTE #	REASON NOTES	ADMIN/ DISPENSED BY:	AMOUNT OF/ WASTE/ HUB LOSS	AMOUNT ADDED	AMOUNT USED	ENDING BALANCE
				☐ BEGINNING BALANCE OR	☐ BALANCE FROM PREVIOUS PAGE ⇧				

CONTROLLED SUBSTANCE: _____ STRENGTH: _____ FROM: _____

DATE	CLIENT, PATIENT	ADDRESS/ID/SERIAL #	UNIQUE BOTTLE #	REASON NOTES	ADMIN/ DISPENSED BY:	AMOUNT OF/ WASTE/ HUB LOSS	AMOUNT ADDED	AMOUNT USED	ENDING BALANCE
				☐ BEGINNING BALANCE OR	☐ BALANCE FROM PREVIOUS PAGE			⇧	

CONTROLLED SUBSTANCE: .... STRENGTH: .... FROM: ....

DATE	CLIENT, PATIENT	ADDRESS/ID/SERIAL #	UNIQUE BOTTLE #	REASON NOTES	ADMIN/ DISPENSED BY:	AMOUNT OF/ WASTE/ HUB LOSS	AMOUNT ADDED	AMOUNT USED	ENDING BALANCE
						☐ BEGINNING BALANCE OR ☐ BALANCE FROM PREVIOUS PAGE ⇧				

DATE	CLIENT, PATIENT	ADDRESS/ID/SERIAL #	UNIQUE BOTTLE #	REASON NOTES	ADMIN/ DISPENSED BY:	AMOUNT OF/ WASTE/ HUB LOSS	AMOUNT ADDED	AMOUNT USED	ENDING BALANCE
				☐ BEGINNING BALANCE OR ☐ BALANCE FROM PREVIOUS PAGE ⇧					

CONTROLLED SUBSTANCE: .... STRENGTH: .... FROM: ....

DATE	CLIENT, PATIENT	ADDRESS/ID/SERIAL #	UNIQUE BOTTLE #	REASON NOTES	ADMIN/ DISPENSED BY:	AMOUNT OF/ WASTE/ HUB LOSS	AMOUNT ADDED	AMOUNT USED	ENDING BALANCE
				☐ BEGINNING BALANCE OR		☐ BALANCE FROM PREVIOUS PAGE		⇧	

CONTROLLED SUBSTANCE:

STRENGTH:

DATE	CLIENT, PATIENT	ADDRESS/ID/SERIAL #	UNIQUE BOTTLE #	REASON NOTES	ADMIN/ DISPENSED BY:	AMOUNT OF/ WASTE/ HUB LOSS	AMOUNT ADDED	AMOUNT USED	ENDING BALANCE
				☐ BEGINNING BALANCE OR	☐ BALANCE FROM PREVIOUS PAGE			⇧	

CONTROLLED SUBSTANCE: .... STRENGTH: .... FROM: ....

DATE	CLIENT, PATIENT	ADDRESS/ID/SERIAL #	UNIQUE BOTTLE #	REASON NOTES	ADMIN/ DISPENSED BY:	AMOUNT OF/ WASTE/ HUB LOSS	AMOUNT ADDED	AMOUNT USED	ENDING BALANCE
				□ BEGINNING BALANCE OR		□ BALANCE FROM PREVIOUS PAGE ⇧			

DATE	CLIENT, PATIENT	ADDRESS/ID/SERIAL #	UNIQUE BOTTE #	REASON NOTES	ADMIN/ DISPENSED BY:	AMOUNT OF/ WASTE/ HUB LOSS	AMOUNT ADDED	AMOUNT USED	ENDING BALANCE
				☐ BEGINNING BALANCE OR ☐ BALANCE FROM PREVIOUS PAGE				⇧	

CONTROLLED SUBSTANCE: ....

STRENGTH: ....   FROM: ....

DATE	CLIENT, PATIENT	ADDRESS/ID/SERIAL #	UNIQUE BOTTLE #	REASON NOTES	ADMIN/ DISPENSED BY:	AMOUNT OF/ WASTE/ HUB LOSS	AMOUNT ADDED	AMOUNT USED	ENDING BALANCE
				☐ BEGINNING BALANCE OR		☐ BALANCE FROM PREVIOUS PAGE		⬆	

CONTROLLED SUBSTANCE:

STRENGTH:

FROM:

DATE	CLIENT, PATIENT	ADDRESS/ID/SERIAL #	UNIQUE BOTTLE #	REASON NOTES	ADMIN/ DISPENSED BY:	AMOUNT OF/ WASTE/ HUB LOSS	AMOUNT ADDED	AMOUNT USED	ENDING BALANCE
						☐ BEGINNING BALANCE OR ☐ BALANCE FROM PREVIOUS PAGE ⇧			

CONTROLLED SUBSTANCE: .... STRENGTH: .... FROM: ....

DATE	CLIENT, PATIENT	ADDRESS/ID/SERIAL #	UNIQUE BOTTE #	REASON NOTES	ADMIN/ DISPENSED BY:	AMOUNT OF/ WASTE/ HUB LOSS	AMOUNT ADDED	AMOUNT USED	ENDING BALANCE
				☐ BEGINNING BALANCE OR		☐ BALANCE FROM PREVIOUS PAGE		⇧	

DATE	CLIENT, PATIENT	ADDRESS/ID/SERIAL #	UNIQUE BOTTLE #	REASON NOTES	ADMIN/ DISPENSED BY:	AMOUNT OF/ WASTE/ HUB LOSS	AMOUNT ADDED	AMOUNT USED	ENDING BALANCE
				☐ BEGINNING BALANCE OR ☐ BALANCE FROM PREVIOUS PAGE ⬆					

CONTROLLED SUBSTANCE: .... STRENGTH: .... FROM: ....

DATE	CLIENT, PATIENT	ADDRESS/ID/SERIAL #	UNIQUE BOTTLE #	REASON NOTES	ADMIN/ DISPENSED BY:	AMOUNT OF/ WASTE/ HUB LOSS	AMOUNT ADDED	AMOUNT USED	ENDING BALANCE
				☐ BEGINNING BALANCE OR		☐ BALANCE FROM PREVIOUS PAGE		⬆	

CONTROLLED SUBSTANCE: .... STRENGTH: ....

DATE	CLIENT, PATIENT	ADDRESS/ID/SERIAL #	UNIQUE BOTTLE #	REASON NOTES	ADMIN/ DISPENSED BY:	AMOUNT OF/ WASTE/ HUB LOSS	AMOUNT ADDED	AMOUNT USED	ENDING BALANCE
	☐ BEGINNING BALANCE OR ☐ BALANCE FROM PREVIOUS PAGE ⇧								

CONTROLLED SUBSTANCE: .... STRENGTH: .... FROM: ....

DATE	CLIENT, PATIENT	ADDRESS/ID/SERIAL #	UNIQUE BOTTE #	REASON NOTES	ADMIN/ DISPENSED BY:	AMOUNT OF/ WASTE/ HUB LOSS	AMOUNT ADDED	AMOUNT USED	ENDING BALANCE
				☐ BEGINNING BALANCE OR		☐ BALANCE FROM PREVIOUS PAGE ⇧			

DATE	CLIENT, PATIENT	ADDRESS/ID/SERIAL #	UNIQUE BOTTE #	REASON NOTES	ADMIN/ DISPENSED BY:	AMOUNT OF/ WASTE/ HUB LOSS	AMOUNT ADDED	AMOUNT USED	ENDING BALANCE
				☐ BEGINNING BALANCE OR		☐ BALANCE FROM PREVIOUS PAGE		⇧	

CONTROLLED SUBSTANCE: ....

STRENGTH: .... FROM: ....

DATE	CLIENT, PATIENT	ADDRESS/ID/SERIAL #	UNIQUE BOTTLE #	REASON NOTES	ADMIN/ DISPENSED BY:	AMOUNT OF/ WASTE/ HUB LOSS	AMOUNT ADDED	AMOUNT USED	ENDING BALANCE
				☐ BEGINNING BALANCE OR		☐ BALANCE FROM PREVIOUS PAGE		⇧	

CONTROLLED SUBSTANCE:

STRENGTH:

FROM:

DATE	CLIENT, PATIENT	ADDRESS/ID/SERIAL #	UNIQUE BOTTLE #	REASON NOTES	ADMIN/ DISPENSED BY:	AMOUNT OF/ WASTE/ HUB LOSS	AMOUNT ADDED	AMOUNT USED	ENDING BALANCE
				☐ BEGINNING BALANCE OR		☐ BALANCE FROM PREVIOUS PAGE		⇧	

CONTROLLED SUBSTANCE: ....   STRENGTH: ....   FROM: ....

DATE	CLIENT, PATIENT	ADDRESS/ID/SERIAL #	UNIQUE BOTTE #	REASON NOTES	ADMIN/ DISPENSED BY:	AMOUNT OF/ WASTE/ HUB LOSS	AMOUNT ADDED	AMOUNT USED	ENDING BALANCE
				☐ BEGINNING BALANCE OR		☐ BALANCE FROM PREVIOUS PAGE		⇧	

DATE	CLIENT, PATIENT	ADDRESS/ID/SERIAL #	UNIQUE BOTTE #	REASON NOTES	ADMIN/ DISPENSED BY:	AMOUNT OF/ WASTE/ HUB LOSS	AMOUNT ADDED	AMOUNT USED	ENDING BALANCE
				☐ BEGINNING BALANCE OR	☐ BALANCE FROM PREVIOUS PAGE			⇧	

CONTROLLED SUBSTANCE: ....

STRENGTH: ....

FROM: ....

DATE	CLIENT, PATIENT	ADDRESS/ID/SERIAL #	UNIQUE BOTTE #	REASON NOTES	ADMIN/ DISPENSED BY:	AMOUNT OF/ WASTE/ HUB LOSS	AMOUNT ADDED	AMOUNT USED	ENDING BALANCE
				☐ BEGINNING BALANCE OR	☐ BALANCE FROM PREVIOUS PAGE			⇧	

CONTROLLED SUBSTANCE

DATE	CLIENT, PATIENT	ADDRESS/ID/SERIAL #	UNIQUE BOTTLE #	REASON NOTES	ADMIN/ DISPENSED BY:	AMOUNT OF/ WASTE/ HUB LOSS	AMOUNT ADDED	AMOUNT USED	ENDING BALANCE
				☐ BEGINNING BALANCE OR		☐ BALANCE FROM PREVIOUS PAGE			

CONTROLLED SUBSTANCE: .... STRENGTH: .... FROM: ....

DATE	CLIENT, PATIENT	ADDRESS/ID/SERIAL #	UNIQUE BOTTLE #	REASON NOTES	ADMIN/ DISPENSED BY:	AMOUNT OF/ WASTE/ HUB LOSS	AMOUNT ADDED	AMOUNT USED	ENDING BALANCE
				☐ BEGINNING BALANCE OR		☐ BALANCE FROM PREVIOUS PAGE		⇧	

DATE	CLIENT, PATIENT	ADDRESS/ID/SERIAL #	UNIQUE BOTTLE #	REASON NOTES	ADMIN/ DISPENSED BY:	AMOUNT OF/ WASTE/ HUB LOSS	AMOUNT ADDED	AMOUNT USED	ENDING BALANCE
				☐ BEGINNING BALANCE OR		☐ BALANCE FROM PREVIOUS PAGE		⇦	

CONTROLLED SUBSTANCE: _____   STRENGTH: _____   FROM: _____

DATE	CLIENT, PATIENT	ADDRESS/ID/SERIAL #	UNIQUE BOTTLE #	REASON NOTES	ADMIN/ DISPENSED BY:	AMOUNT OF/ WASTE/ HUB LOSS	AMOUNT ADDED	AMOUNT USED	ENDING BALANCE
				☐ BEGINNING BALANCE OR	☐ BALANCE FROM PREVIOUS PAGE			⇧	

DATE	CLIENT, PATIENT	ADDRESS/ID/SERIAL #	UNIQUE BOTTE #	REASON NOTES	ADMIN/ DISPENSED BY:	AMOUNT OF/ WASTE/ HUB LOSS	AMOUNT ADDED	AMOUNT USED	ENDING BALANCE
				☐ BEGINNING BALANCE OR ☐ BALANCE FROM PREVIOUS PAGE				⬆	

CONTROLLED SUBSTANCE: .... STRENGTH: .... FROM: ....

DATE	CLIENT, PATIENT	ADDRESS/ID/SERIAL #	UNIQUE BOTTLE #	REASON NOTES	ADMIN/ DISPENSED BY:	AMOUNT OF/ WASTE/ HUB LOSS	AMOUNT ADDED	AMOUNT USED	ENDING BALANCE
						☐ BEGINNING BALANCE OR	☐ BALANCE FROM PREVIOUS PAGE	⇧	

DATE	CLIENT, PATIENT	ADDRESS/ID/SERIAL #	UNIQUE BOTTE #	REASON NOTES	ADMIN/ DISPENSED BY:	AMOUNT OF/ WASTE/ HUB LOSS	AMOUNT ADDED	AMOUNT USED	ENDING BALANCE
				☐ BEGINNING BALANCE OR	☐ BALANCE FROM PREVIOUS PAGE ⇧				

CONTROLLED SUBSTANCE: .... STRENGTH: .... FROM: ....

DATE	CLIENT, PATIENT	ADDRESS/ID/SERIAL #	UNIQUE BOTTE #	REASON NOTES	ADMIN/ DISPENSED BY:	AMOUNT OF/ WASTE/ HUB LOSS	AMOUNT ADDED	AMOUNT USED	ENDING BALANCE
				☐ BEGINNING BALANCE OR		☐ BALANCE FROM PREVIOUS PAGE		⇧	

CONTROLLED SUBSTANCE: _____

STRENGTH: _____

FROM: _____

DATE	CLIENT, PATIENT	ADDRESS/ID/SERIAL #	UNIQUE BOTTE #	REASON NOTES	ADMIN/ DISPENSED BY:	AMOUNT OF/ WASTE/ HUB LOSS	AMOUNT ADDED	AMOUNT USED	ENDING BALANCE
				☐ BEGINNING BALANCE OR		☐ BALANCE FROM PREVIOUS PAGE ⇧			

CONTROLLED SUBSTANCE: .... STRENGTH: .... FROM: ....

DATE	CLIENT, PATIENT	ADDRESS/ID/SERIAL #	UNIQUE BOTTE #	REASON NOTES	ADMIN/ DISPENSED BY:	AMOUNT OF/ WASTE/ HUB LOSS	AMOUNT ADDED	AMOUNT USED	ENDING BALANCE
				☐ BEGINNING BALANCE OR		☐ BALANCE FROM PREVIOUS PAGE		⇧	

DATE	CLIENT, PATIENT	ADDRESS/ID/SERIAL #	UNIQUE BOTTE #	REASON NOTES	ADMIN/ DISPENSED BY:	AMOUNT OF/ WASTE/ HUB LOSS	AMOUNT ADDED	AMOUNT USED	ENDING BALANCE
						☐ BEGINNING BALANCE OR	☐ BALANCE FROM PREVIOUS PAGE	⇧	

CONTROLLED SUBSTANCE: .... STRENGTH: .... FROM: ....

DATE	CLIENT, PATIENT	ADDRESS/ID/SERIAL #	UNIQUE BOTTLE #	REASON NOTES	ADMIN/ DISPENSED BY:	AMOUNT OF/ WASTE/ HUB LOSS	AMOUNT ADDED	AMOUNT USED	ENDING BALANCE
				☐ BEGINNING BALANCE OR		☐ BALANCE FROM PREVIOUS PAGE ⇧			

DATE	CLIENT, PATIENT	ADDRESS/ID/SERIAL #	UNIQUE BOTTLE #	REASON NOTES	ADMIN/ DISPENSED BY:	AMOUNT OF/ WASTE/ HUB LOSS	AMOUNT ADDED	AMOUNT USED	ENDING BALANCE
				☐ BEGINNING BALANCE OR		☐ BALANCE FROM PREVIOUS PAGE		⇧	

CONTROLLED SUBSTANCE: .... STRENGTH: .... FROM: ....

DATE	CLIENT, PATIENT	ADDRESS/ID/SERIAL #	UNIQUE BOTTLE #	REASON NOTES	ADMIN/ DISPENSED BY:	AMOUNT OF/ WASTE/ HUB LOSS	AMOUNT ADDED	AMOUNT USED	ENDING BALANCE
				☐ BEGINNING BALANCE OR	☐ BALANCE FROM PREVIOUS PAGE			⇧	

DATE	CLIENT, PATIENT	ADDRESS/ID/SERIAL #	UNIQUE BOTTE #	REASON NOTES	ADMIN/ DISPENSED BY:	AMOUNT OF/ WASTE/ HUB LOSS	AMOUNT ADDED	AMOUNT USED	ENDING BALANCE
						☐ BALANCE FROM PREVIOUS PAGE ⇧			
					☐ BEGINNING BALANCE OR				

CONTROLLED SUBSTANCE: .... STRENGTH: .... FROM: ....

DATE	CLIENT, PATIENT	ADDRESS/ID/SERIAL #	UNIQUE BOTTE #	REASON NOTES	ADMIN/ DISPENSED BY:	AMOUNT OF/ WASTE/ HUB LOSS	AMOUNT ADDED	AMOUNT USED	ENDING BALANCE
				☐ BEGINNING BALANCE OR		☐ BALANCE FROM PREVIOUS PAGE		⇧	

CONTROLLED SUBSTANCE: _____ STRENGTH: _____ FROM: _____

DATE	CLIENT, PATIENT	ADDRESS/ID/SERIAL #	UNIQUE BOTTLE #	REASON NOTES	ADMIN/ DISPENSED BY:	AMOUNT OF/ WASTE/ HUB LOSS	AMOUNT ADDED	AMOUNT USED	ENDING BALANCE
				☐ BEGINNING BALANCE OR		☐ BALANCE FROM PREVIOUS PAGE		⇧	

CONTROLLED SUBSTANCE: .... STRENGTH: .... FROM: ....

DATE	CLIENT, PATIENT	ADDRESS/I.D/SERIAL #	UNIQUE BOTTLE #	REASON NOTES	ADMIN/ DISPENSED BY:	AMOUNT OF/ WASTE/ HUB LOSS	AMOUNT ADDED	AMOUNT USED	ENDING BALANCE
				☐ BEGINNING BALANCE OR		☐ BALANCE FROM PREVIOUS PAGE		⇧	

DATE	CLIENT, PATIENT	ADDRESS/ID/SERIAL #	UNIQUE BOTTE #	REASON NOTES	ADMIN/ DISPENSED BY:	AMOUNT OF/ WASTE/ HUB LOSS	AMOUNT ADDED	AMOUNT USED	ENDING BALANCE
				☐ BEGINNING BALANCE OR		☐ BALANCE FROM PREVIOUS PAGE		⇧	

CONTROLLED SUBSTANCE: _____   STRENGTH: _____   FROM: _____

DATE	CLIENT, PATIENT	ADDRESS/ID/SERIAL #	UNIQUE BOTTLE #	REASON NOTES	ADMIN/ DISPENSED BY:	AMOUNT OF/ WASTE/ HUB LOSS	AMOUNT ADDED	AMOUNT USED	ENDING BALANCE
				☐ BEGINNING BALANCE OR		☐ BALANCE FROM PREVIOUS PAGE		⇧	

CONTROLLED SUBSTANCE: .... STRENGTH: .... FROM: ....

DATE	CLIENT. PATIENT	ADDRESS/ID/SERIAL #	UNIQUE BOTTE #	REASON NOTES	ADMIN/ DISPENSED BY:	AMOUNT OF/ WASTE/ HUB LOSS	AMOUNT ADDED	AMOUNT USED	ENDING BALANCE
				☐ BEGINNING BALANCE OR ☐ BALANCE FROM PREVIOUS PAGE				⇧	

CONTROLLED SUBSTANCE: .... STRENGTH: .... FROM: ....

DATE	CLIENT, PATIENT	ADDRESS/ID/SERIAL #	UNIQUE BOTTLE #	REASON NOTES	ADMIN/ DISPENSED BY:	AMOUNT OF/ WASTE/ HUB LOSS	AMOUNT ADDED	AMOUNT USED	ENDING BALANCE
				☐ BEGINNING BALANCE OR		☐ BALANCE FROM PREVIOUS PAGE		⇧	

DATE	CLIENT, PATIENT	ADDRESS/ID/SERIAL #	UNIQUE BOTTE #	REASON NOTES	ADMIN/ DISPENSED BY:	AMOUNT OF/ WASTE/ HUB LOSS	AMOUNT ADDED	AMOUNT USED	ENDING BALANCE
				☐ BEGINNING BALANCE OR ☐ BALANCE FROM PREVIOUS PAGE ⇧					

CONTROLLED SUBSTANCE: .... STRENGTH: .... FROM: ....

DATE	CLIENT, PATIENT	ADDRESS/ID/SERIAL #	UNIQUE BOTTLE #	REASON NOTES	ADMIN/ DISPENSED BY:	AMOUNT OF/ WASTE/ HUB LOSS	AMOUNT ADDED	AMOUNT USED	ENDING BALANCE
				☐ BEGINNING BALANCE OR		☐ BALANCE FROM PREVIOUS PAGE		⇧	

CONTROLLED SUBSTANCE: _____ STRENGTH: _____ FROM: _____

DATE	CLIENT, PATIENT	ADDRESS/ID/SERIAL #	UNIQUE BOTTLE #	REASON NOTES	ADMIN/ DISPENSED BY:	AMOUNT OF/ WASTE/ HUB LOSS	AMOUNT ADDED	AMOUNT USED	ENDING BALANCE
				☐ BEGINNING BALANCE OR		☐ BALANCE FROM PREVIOUS PAGE		⇧	

CONTROLLED SUBSTANCE: - - - - - - - - - -   STRENGTH: - - - - - - - - - -   FROM: - - - - - - - - - -

DATE	CLIENT, PATIENT	ADDRESS/ID/SERIAL #	UNIQUE BOTTLE #	REASON NOTES	ADMIN/ DISPENSED BY:	AMOUNT OF/ WASTE/ HUB LOSS	AMOUNT ADDED	AMOUNT USED	ENDING BALANCE
				☐ BEGINNING BALANCE OR		☐ BALANCE FROM PREVIOUS PAGE		⇧	

DATE	CLIENT, PATIENT	ADDRESS/ID/SERIAL #	UNIQUE BOTTE #	REASON NOTES	ADMIN/ DISPENSED BY:	AMOUNT OF/ WASTE/ HUB LOSS	AMOUNT ADDED	AMOUNT USED	ENDING BALANCE
				☐ BEGINNING BALANCE OR		☐ BALANCE FROM PREVIOUS PAGE		⇧	

CONTROLLED SUBSTANCE: .... STRENGTH: .... FROM: ....

DATE	CLIENT, PATIENT	ADDRESS/ID/SERIAL #	UNIQUE BOTTLE #	REASON NOTES	ADMIN/ DISPENSED BY:	AMOUNT OF/ WASTE/ HUB LOSS	AMOUNT ADDED	AMOUNT USED	ENDING BALANCE
				☐ BEGINNING BALANCE OR		☐ BALANCE FROM PREVIOUS PAGE		⇧	

DATE	CLIENT, PATIENT	ADDRESS/ID/SERIAL #	UNIQUE BOTTE #	REASON NOTES	ADMIN/ DISPENSED BY:	AMOUNT OF/ WASTE/ HUB LOSS	AMOUNT ADDED	AMOUNT USED	ENDING BALANCE
				☐ BEGINNING BALANCE OR	☐ BALANCE FROM PREVIOUS PAGE ⇧				

CONTROLLED SUBSTANCE: .... STRENGTH: .... FROM: ....

DATE	CLIENT, PATIENT	ADDRESS/ID/SERIAL #	UNIQUE BOTTE #	REASON NOTES	ADMIN/ DISPENSED BY.	AMOUNT OF/ WASTE/ HUB LOSS	AMOUNT ADDED	AMOUNT USED	ENDING BALANCE
				☐ BEGINNING BALANCE OR		☐ BALANCE FROM PREVIOUS PAGE		⇧	

DATE	CLIENT, PATIENT	ADDRESS/ID/SERIAL #	UNIQUE BOTTE #	REASON NOTES	ADMIN/ DISPENSED BY:	AMOUNT OF/ WASTE/ HUB LOSS	AMOUNT ADDED	AMOUNT USED	ENDING BALANCE
				☐ BEGINNING BALANCE OR ☐ BALANCE FROM PREVIOUS PAGE ⇧					

CONTROLLED SUBSTANCE: .... STRENGTH: .... FROM: ....

DATE	CLIENT, PATIENT	ADDRESS/ID/SERIAL #	UNIQUE BOTTLE #	REASON NOTES	ADMIN/ DISPENSED BY:	AMOUNT OF/ WASTE/ HUB LOSS	AMOUNT ADDED	AMOUNT USED	ENDING BALANCE
				☐ BEGINNING BALANCE OR		☐ BALANCE FROM PREVIOUS PAGE		⇧	

DATE	CLIENT, PATIENT	ADDRESS/ID/SERIAL #	UNIQUE BOTTE #	REASON NOTES	ADMIN/ DISPENSED BY:	AMOUNT OF/ WASTE/ HUB LOSS	AMOUNT ADDED	AMOUNT USED	ENDING BALANCE
				☐ BEGINNING BALANCE OR	☐ BALANCE FROM PREVIOUS PAGE			⇧	

CONTROLLED SUBSTANCE: .... STRENGTH: .... FROM: ....

DATE	CLIENT, PATIENT	ADDRESS/ID/SERIAL #	UNIQUE BOTTLE #	REASON NOTES	ADMIN/ DISPENSED BY:	AMOUNT OF/ WASTE/ HUB LOSS	AMOUNT ADDED	AMOUNT USED	ENDING BALANCE
				☐ BEGINNING BALANCE OR		☐ BALANCE FROM PREVIOUS PAGE ⇧			

DATE	CLIENT, PATIENT	ADDRESS/ID/SERIAL #	UNIQUE BOTTLE #	REASON NOTES	ADMIN/ DISPENSED BY:	AMOUNT OF/ WASTE/ HUB LOSS	AMOUNT ADDED	AMOUNT USED	ENDING BALANCE
				☐ BEGINNING BALANCE OR	☐ BALANCE FROM PREVIOUS PAGE			⇧	

CONTROLLED SUBSTANCE: --------------------- STRENGTH: ----------------------- FROM:

DATE	CLIENT, PATIENT	ADDRESS/ID/SERIAL #	UNIQUE BOTTLE #	REASON NOTES	ADMIN/ DISPENSED BY:	AMOUNT OF/ WASTE/ HUB LOSS	AMOUNT ADDED	AMOUNT USED	ENDING BALANCE
				☐ BEGINNING BALANCE OR		☐ BALANCE FROM PREVIOUS PAGE		⇧	

CONTROLLED SUBSTANCE

DATE	CLIENT, PATIENT	ADDRESS/ID/SERIAL #	UNIQUE BOTTE #	REASON NOTES	ADMIN/ DISPENSED BY:	AMOUNT OF/ WASTE/ HUB LOSS	AMOUNT ADDED	AMOUNT USED	ENDING BALANCE
				□ BEGINNING BALANCE OR		□ BALANCE FROM PREVIOUS PAGE		⇧	

CONTROLLED SUBSTANCE: .... STRENGTH: .... FROM: ....

DATE	CLIENT, PATIENT	ADDRESS/ID/SERIAL #	UNIQUE BOTTLE #	REASON NOTES	ADMIN/ DISPENSED BY:	AMOUNT OF/ WASTE/ HUB LOSS	AMOUNT ADDED	AMOUNT USED	ENDING BALANCE
				☐ BEGINNING BALANCE OR		☐ BALANCE FROM PREVIOUS PAGE		⇧	

DATE	CLIENT, PATIENT	ADDRESS/ID/SERIAL #	UNIQUE BOTTE #	REASON NOTES	ADMIN/ DISPENSED BY:	AMOUNT OF/ WASTE/ HUB LOSS	AMOUNT ADDED	AMOUNT USED	ENDING BALANCE
				☐ BEGINNING BALANCE OR	☐ BALANCE FROM PREVIOUS PAGE			⇧	

CONTROLLED SUBSTANCE: .... STRENGTH: .... FROM: ....

DATE	CLIENT, PATIENT	ADDRESS/ID/SERIAL #	UNIQUE BOTTLE #	REASON NOTES	ADMIN/ DISPENSED BY:	AMOUNT OF/ WASTE/ HUB LOSS	AMOUNT ADDED	AMOUNT USED	ENDING BALANCE
						☐ BEGINNING BALANCE OR	☐ BALANCE FROM PREVIOUS PAGE	⇧	

CONTROLLED SUBSTANCE:

STRENGTH: _____ FROM: _____

DATE	CLIENT, PATIENT	ADDRESS/ID/SERIAL #	UNIQUE BOTTE #	REASON NOTES	ADMIN/ DISPENSED BY:	AMOUNT OF/ WASTE/ HUB LOSS	AMOUNT ADDED	AMOUNT USED	ENDING BALANCE
				☐ BEGINNING BALANCE OR	☐ BALANCE FROM PREVIOUS PAGE			⇧	

CONTROLLED SUBSTANCE: ....   STRENGTH: ....   FROM: ....

DATE	CLIENT, PATIENT	ADDRESS/ID/SERIAL #	UNIQUE BOTTLE #	REASON NOTES	ADMIN/ DISPENSED BY:	AMOUNT OF/ WASTE/ HUB LOSS	AMOUNT ADDED	AMOUNT USED	ENDING BALANCE
				☐ BEGINNING BALANCE OR		☐ BALANCE FROM PREVIOUS PAGE		⇧	

DATE	CLIENT, PATIENT	ADDRESS/ID/SERIAL #	UNIQUE BOTTE #	REASON NOTES	ADMIN/ DISPENSED BY:	AMOUNT OF/ WASTE/ HUB LOSS	AMOUNT ADDED	AMOUNT USED	ENDING BALANCE
				☐ BEGINNING BALANCE OR		☐ BALANCE FROM PREVIOUS PAGE		⇧	

CONTROLLED SUBSTANCE: .... STRENGTH: .... FROM: ....

DATE	CLIENT, PATIENT	ADDRESS/ID/SERIAL #	UNIQUE BOTTLE #	REASON NOTES	ADMIN/ DISPENSED BY:	AMOUNT OF/ WASTE/ HUB LOSS	AMOUNT ADDED	AMOUNT USED	ENDING BALANCE
				☐ BEGINNING BALANCE OR		☐ BALANCE FROM PREVIOUS PAGE		⇧	

DATE	CLIENT, PATIENT	ADDRESS/ID/SERIAL #	UNIQUE BOTTLE #	REASON NOTES	ADMIN/ DISPENSED BY:	AMOUNT OF/ WASTE/ HUB LOSS	AMOUNT ADDED	AMOUNT USED	ENDING BALANCE
				☐ BEGINNING BALANCE OR		☐ BALANCE FROM PREVIOUS PAGE		⇧	

CONTROLLED SUBSTANCE: .... STRENGTH: .... FROM: ....

DATE	CLIENT, PATIENT	ADDRESS/ID/SERIAL #	UNIQUE BOTTLE #	REASON NOTES	ADMIN/ DISPENSED BY:	AMOUNT OF/ WASTE/ HUB LOSS	AMOUNT ADDED	AMOUNT USED	ENDING BALANCE
				☐ BEGINNING BALANCE OR		☐ BALANCE FROM PREVIOUS PAGE		⇧	

DATE	CLIENT, PATIENT	ADDRESS/ID/SERIAL #	UNIQUE BOTTLE #	REASON NOTES	ADMIN/ DISPENSED BY:	AMOUNT OF/ WASTE/ HUB LOSS	AMOUNT ADDED	AMOUNT USED	ENDING BALANCE
				☐ BEGINNING BALANCE OR	☐ BALANCE FROM PREVIOUS PAGE			⇧	

CONTROLLED SUBSTANCE: .... STRENGTH: .... FROM: ....

DATE	CLIENT, PATIENT	ADDRESS/ID/SERIAL #	UNIQUE BOTTE #	REASON NOTES	ADMIN/ DISPENSED BY:	AMOUNT OF/ WASTE/ HUB LOSS	AMOUNT ADDED	AMOUNT USED	ENDING BALANCE
				☐ BEGINNING BALANCE OR		☐ BALANCE FROM PREVIOUS PAGE		⇧	

DATE	CLIENT, PATIENT	ADDRESS/ID/SERIAL #	UNIQUE BOTTLE #	REASON NOTES	ADMIN/ DISPENSED BY:	AMOUNT OF/ WASTE/ HUB LOSS	AMOUNT ADDED	AMOUNT USED	ENDING BALANCE
				☐ BEGINNING BALANCE OR	☐ BALANCE FROM PREVIOUS PAGE			⇧	

CONTROLLED SUBSTANCE: .... STRENGTH: .... FROM: ....

DATE	CLIENT, PATIENT	ADDRESS/ID/SERIAL #	UNIQUE BOTTE #	REASON NOTES	ADMIN/ DISPENSED BY.	AMOUNT OF/ WASTE/ HUB LOSS	AMOUNT ADDED	AMOUNT USED	ENDING BALANCE
			☐ BEGINNING BALANCE OR	☐ BALANCE FROM PREVIOUS PAGE				⇧	

DATE	CLIENT, PATIENT	ADDRESS/ID/SERIAL #	UNIQUE BOTTLE #	REASON NOTES	ADMIN/ DISPENSED BY:	AMOUNT OF/ WASTE/ HUB LOSS	AMOUNT ADDED	AMOUNT USED	ENDING BALANCE
				□ BEGINNING BALANCE OR		□ BALANCE FROM PREVIOUS PAGE		⇧	

CONTROLLED SUBSTANCE: .... STRENGTH: .... FROM: ....

DATE	CLIENT, PATIENT	ADDRESS/ID/SERIAL #	UNIQUE BOTTLE #	REASON NOTES	ADMIN/ DISPENSED BY:	AMOUNT OF/ WASTE/ HUB LOSS	AMOUNT ADDED	AMOUNT USED	ENDING BALANCE
				☐ BEGINNING BALANCE OR		☐ BALANCE FROM PREVIOUS PAGE		⇧	

CONTROLLED SUBSTANCE:............ STRENGTH:...........

DATE	CLIENT, PATIENT	ADDRESS/ID/SERIAL #	UNIQUE BOTTE #	REASON NOTES	ADMIN/ DISPENSED BY:	AMOUNT OF/ WASTE/ HUB LOSS	AMOUNT ADDED	AMOUNT USED	ENDING BALANCE
				☐ BEGINNING BALANCE OR		☐ BALANCE FROM PREVIOUS PAGE		⬆	

CONTROLLED SUBSTANCE: .... STRENGTH: .... FROM: ....

DATE	CLIENT, PATIENT	ADDRESS/ID/SERIAL #	UNIQUE BOTTE #	REASON NOTES	ADMIN/ DISPENSED BY:	AMOUNT OF/ WASTE/ HUB LOSS	AMOUNT ADDED	AMOUNT USED	ENDING BALANCE
				☐ BEGINNING BALANCE OR ☐ BALANCE FROM PREVIOUS PAGE ⇧					

DATE	CLIENT, PATIENT	ADDRESS/ID/SERIAL #	UNIQUE BOTTLE #	REASON NOTES	ADMIN/ DISPENSED BY:	AMOUNT OF/ WASTE/ HUB LOSS	AMOUNT ADDED	AMOUNT USED	ENDING BALANCE
				☐ BEGINNING BALANCE OR		☐ BALANCE FROM PREVIOUS PAGE		⇧	

CONTROLLED SUBSTANCE: .... STRENGTH: .... FROM: ....

DATE	CLIENT, PATIENT	ADDRESS/ID/SERIAL #	UNIQUE BOTTLE #	REASON NOTES	ADMIN/ DISPENSED BY:	AMOUNT OF/ WASTE/ HUB LOSS	AMOUNT ADDED	AMOUNT USED	ENDING BALANCE
				☐ BEGINNING BALANCE OR		☐ BALANCE FROM PREVIOUS PAGE		⇧	

CONTROLLED SUBSTANCE...

STRENGTH:... FROM:...

DATE	CLIENT, PATIENT	ADDRESS/ID/SERIAL #	UNIQUE BOTTLE #	REASON NOTES	ADMIN/ DISPENSED BY:	AMOUNT OF/ WASTE/ HUB LOSS	AMOUNT ADDED	AMOUNT USED	ENDING BALANCE
				☐ BEGINNING BALANCE OR		☐ BALANCE FROM PREVIOUS PAGE		⇦	

CONTROLLED SUBSTANCE: .... STRENGTH: .... FROM: ....

DATE	CLIENT, PATIENT	ADDRESS/ID/SERIAL #	UNIQUE BOTTE #	REASON NOTES	ADMIN/ DISPENSED BY:	AMOUNT OF/ WASTE/ HUB LOSS	AMOUNT ADDED	AMOUNT USED	ENDING BALANCE
				☐ BEGINNING BALANCE OR		☐ BALANCE FROM PREVIOUS PAGE		⇧	

DATE	CLIENT, PATIENT	ADDRESS/ID/SERIAL #	UNIQUE BOTTLE #	REASON NOTES	ADMIN/ DISPENSED BY:	AMOUNT OF/ WASTE/ HUB LOSS	AMOUNT ADDED	AMOUNT USED	ENDING BALANCE
				☐ BEGINNING BALANCE OR ☐ BALANCE FROM PREVIOUS PAGE ⇧					

CONTROLLED SUBSTANCE: ....   STRENGTH: ....   FROM: ....

DATE	CLIENT, PATIENT	ADDRESS/ID/SERIAL #	UNIQUE BOTTLE #	REASON NOTES	ADMIN/ DISPENSED BY:	AMOUNT OF/ WASTE/ HUB LOSS	AMOUNT ADDED	AMOUNT USED	ENDING BALANCE
				☐ BEGINNING BALANCE OR	☐ BALANCE FROM PREVIOUS PAGE			⇧	

DATE	CLIENT, PATIENT	ADDRESS/ID/SERIAL #	UNIQUE BOTTLE #	REASON NOTES	ADMIN/ DISPENSED BY:	AMOUNT OF/ WASTE/ HUB LOSS	AMOUNT ADDED	AMOUNT USED	ENDING BALANCE
				☐ BEGINNING BALANCE OR	☐ BALANCE FROM PREVIOUS PAGE			⬆	

CONTROLLED SUBSTANCE: .... STRENGTH: .... FROM: ....

DATE	CLIENT, PATIENT	ADDRESS/ID/SERIAL #	UNIQUE BOTTLE #	REASON NOTES	ADMIN/ DISPENSED BY:	AMOUNT OF/ WASTE/ HUB LOSS	AMOUNT ADDED	AMOUNT USED	ENDING BALANCE
				☐ BEGINNING BALANCE OR		☐ BALANCE FROM PREVIOUS PAGE		⇧	

DATE	CLIENT, PATIENT	ADDRESS/ID/SERIAL #	UNIQUE BOTTLE #	REASON NOTES	ADMIN/ DISPENSED BY:	AMOUNT OF/ WASTE/ HUB LOSS	AMOUNT ADDED	AMOUNT USED	ENDING BALANCE
				☐ BEGINNING BALANCE OR		☐ BALANCE FROM PREVIOUS PAGE		⇧	

CONTROLLED SUBSTANCE: .... STRENGTH: .... FROM: ....

DATE	CLIENT, PATIENT	ADDRESS/ID/SERIAL #	UNIQUE BOTTE #	REASON NOTES	ADMIN/ DISPENSED BY:	AMOUNT OF/ WASTE/ HUB LOSS	AMOUNT ADDED	AMOUNT USED	ENDING BALANCE
				☐ BEGINNING BALANCE OR		☐ BALANCE FROM PREVIOUS PAGE		⬆	

DATE	CLIENT, PATIENT	ADDRESS/ID/SERIAL #	UNIQUE BOTTLE #	REASON NOTES	ADMIN/ DISPENSED BY:	AMOUNT OF/ WASTE/ HUB LOSS	AMOUNT ADDED	AMOUNT USED	ENDING BALANCE
						☐ BEGINNING BALANCE OR ☐ BALANCE FROM PREVIOUS PAGE ⬆			

CONTROLLED SUBSTANCE: .... STRENGTH: .... FROM: ....

DATE	CLIENT, PATIENT ADDRESS/ID/SERIAL #	UNIQUE BOTTE #	REASON NOTES	ADMIN/ DISPENSED BY:	AMOUNT OF/ WASTE/ HUB LOSS	AMOUNT ADDED	AMOUNT USED	ENDING BALANCE
			☐ BEGINNING BALANCE OR		☐ BALANCE FROM PREVIOUS PAGE ⇧			

DATE	CLIENT, PATIENT	ADDRESS/ID/SERIAL #	UNIQUE BOTTE #	REASON NOTES	ADMIN/ DISPENSED BY:	AMOUNT OF/ WASTE/ HUB LOSS	AMOUNT ADDED	AMOUNT USED	ENDING BALANCE
				☐ BEGINNING BALANCE OR		☐ BALANCE FROM PREVIOUS PAGE ⬆			

CONTROLLED SUBSTANCE: .... STRENGTH: .... FROM: ....

DATE	CLIENT, PATIENT	ADDRESS/ID/SERIAL #	UNIQUE BOTTLE #	REASON NOTES	ADMIN/ DISPENSED BY:	AMOUNT OF/ WASTE/ HUB LOSS	AMOUNT ADDED	AMOUNT USED	ENDING BALANCE
				☐ BEGINNING BALANCE OR		☐ BALANCE FROM PREVIOUS PAGE		⇧	

CONTROLLED SUBSTANCE: _____ STRENGTH: _____ FROM: _____

DATE	CLIENT, PATIENT	ADDRESS/ID/SERIAL #	UNIQUE BOTTLE #	REASON NOTES	ADMIN/ DISPENSED BY:	AMOUNT OF/ WASTE/ HUB LOSS	AMOUNT ADDED	AMOUNT USED	ENDING BALANCE
				☐ BEGINNING BALANCE OR		☐ BALANCE FROM PREVIOUS PAGE		⇧	

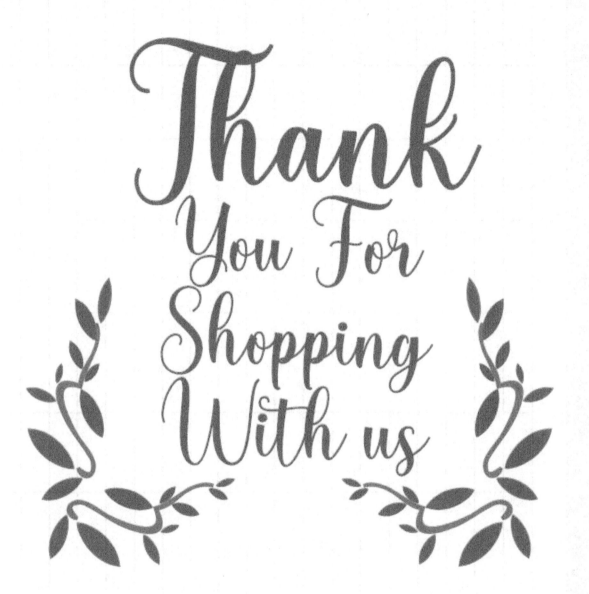

Thank you

for purchasing our products on Amazon.

We strive to offer you the best value and service possible.

Please take a moment to rate us as a seller on the Amazon.

Made in the USA
Las Vegas, NV
27 December 2024

15469055R00070